Start Talking: Intimacy

A Couples' Guide to Discussing Sex:
A Professional Viewpoint from
a Biblical Perspective

Melissa Hague, M.D.
Neil Hague
James A. Smith, LCMFT
Julie Smith

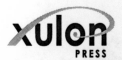

xulon
PRESS

Start Talking: Intimacy
A Couples' Guide to Discussing Sex: A Professional Viewpoint
from a Biblical Perspective
by Melissa Hague, M.D. Neil Hague James A. Smith, LCMFT Julie Smith

Printed in the United States of America.

Edited by Xulon Press

ISBN 9781498447157

www.xulonpress.com

Table of Contents

Introduction

I knock on the door and announce, "Hel-low," as I walk in and quickly shut the door behind me. The woman is a beautiful, young 30-something whom I have seen every year for several years. She sits there nervously, the only item of her own wardrobe on her feet in the form of yellow and black striped socks. A sheet lies over her lap, and a gown rests on her shoulders. The exam table is green, with that dreaded crinkly-white paper pulled over it. No doubt, it will not be intact when she leaves, as nervous sweating causes the paper to stick to her skin and become a shredded mess.

I start the usual discussion, "How are you? The kids? The job?" as I examine her thyroid. I listen to her heart and lungs, and then ask her to lie back. As I begin the breast exam (one of the most nerve-wracking parts for any woman with an intact nervous system), I ask the more important questions: "Are you sexually active? Does it hurt? Are you able to orgasm?" I want to gather all the information needed to finish the sensitive exam.

This year, tears brim in her eyes, and she exclaims, "I can't seem to do it anymore." I have heard this before, and though the reasons tend to vary slightly, they have common themes: Too busy, too tired, too many things more important than connecting sexually with the significant other, too painful, too depressed.

After seeing so many women like this, I started to look through the medical literature, searching for an answer to decreased sex drive. That was early in my career, before I realized that "low libido" was truly a symptom of some greater issue. Often, women would have medications that caused a problem, pain with intercourse, decreased sensation, a history of sexual trauma, or a myriad of other issues that led to "decreased sex drive." Until I could figure out a way to help them address these other issues, as well as communicate honestly and effectively with their husbands, I would not be able to address their libido in a manner that was meaningful.

I started to feel ineffective. There are few medical sources for most of the problems I was encountering in the office. There was also the problem that I was only seeing half of the equation (the woman), with the other—and often more complex—part of the equation (the man) missing. I would often have a discussion with women about sex, priorities, pressures, and they would usually say, "I wish my husband was here. I just can't seem to talk to him about this stuff on my own."

Realizing the impracticality of couples' counseling sessions in a busy gynecology office (and my lack of education in this arena), I started looking for resources to help couples have the conversations they needed to get their love life on track. There was a paucity of sex-help books, and some great volumes written by much more qualified individuals than I on how Christians could improve their love life. There was not, however, a simple book with simple questions that could lead to deep conversations and more meaningful intimacy.

Truth be told, I wrote this book more for men who love their wives and want to discuss the issue of intimacy so that they can grow deeper in love. I realize that many women can read volumes on a subject and walk away having a greater depth of knowledge, whereas many men are bored or asleep by page two. The chapters in this book are short and meant to be read out loud together, preferably while in bed. The reading is merely a spring board for the discussion that is to follow. Some of the questions are superficial and some go deeper, but all are meant to help you and your spouse know one another (in the biblical sense) and have a more satisfying connection.

This book is not a substitute for medical consultation or professional counseling. It is simply designed to help you and your spouse have open communication about a variety of issues that can affect your sex life. If you find you have concerns that you cannot resolve with communication and patience, please seek help from a qualified professional.

1.

Awkward

How would I describe the conversations I have had with women about their sex lives? Awkward. Even after many years as a gynecologist, it can be a difficult conversation to have. I once had a friend struggling with sexual issues in her marriage, and she went out of town to find a counselor whom she would never run into, who was not in her church or circle of friends. This confused me, as many of my friends are my patients. I was also a little offended that she would think the counselors in our town were not professional enough to talk in the office on Monday and sing in the choir with her on Sunday. She explained to me that it was just too "awkward" to talk about sex with someone she knew.

Unfortunately, many husbands and wives feel the same way about discussing sex, even in the privacy of their own bedroom. He doesn't want to offend her or make her mad by asking why she doesn't want to have sex. She doesn't want to hurt his feelings by telling him it hurts when they have intercourse. These fears lead to tension and tension leads to...well, silence. I have cared for women who have not had sex with their husbands for months, or even years and it often started with a bad sexual encounter that they never discussed, a period of illness that prevented intimacy, or a harsh word at the wrong time that bred resentment.

So, how *do* you talk about sex? I often tell my patients that you have to say what you are thinking, even if you fear an awkward silence or negative response. You say things in love, with the plan and hope for restoration of intimacy, and you have grace for your lover. You try to leave offense at the door – both speech that would offend your spouse, and your own ability to become offended. You remind yourself that you said "I do" to every part of being married, including intimacy. You "take the plunge" because your lover is worth it, you are worth it, and God intended for you to enjoy one another sexually.

As a reminder, remember that God knows all about sex – He created it! While it may feel weird to pray about sex, Christians often pray about other aspects of life – finances, career, health, etc.—and great intimacy with your spouse is important. Try to pray together, asking God to help you as you start the journey of communication about sex together. Prayer does not have to be complex, fancy, or long. Just start the conversation with God.

Questions

1. What conversations did you and your parents or family have about sex when you were growing up?
2. What was your perception, prior to marriage, of what sex would be like in a married relationship?
3. What is one misconception you had about sex that you wish you would have known to be false?
4. What quality about your spouse do you appreciate the most?
5. Turn to your partner and compliment him or her. Tell your spouse about something he does that provides you with sexual satisfaction, or a part of her body that turns you on.

2.

Is It Really *that* Important?

There are many red flags that I hear when discussing sex with my patients. Perhaps one of the most bothersome to me is when patients who are married say that they are not sexually active because sex is "not important" to them. I usually start with the question, "Not important to whom?" and discover that they have not had a sexual encounter in quite some time. They have made the assumption that sex is not important to their spouse, or that the subject is too much to cover, too painful, or too difficult to resolve. Often, it is actually that it is not important to the wife or its importance has dwindled. All further conversation has stopped regarding the absence of sexual activity. In other cases, the man may have even indicated in conversations that sex isn't important to him anymore, either. The reality is often that the man does not want his wife to feel bad about her lack of sexual desire, or worse, has given up entirely on their sex life.

Such reactions, though, disregard the reality that sex is a vital part of marriage! It is part of God's plan. Through sex, married couples can experience a deeper intimacy that leads to a healthier relationship. It can be a lot fun as well!

The apostle Paul counseled not to abstain from sexual relations except in times of prayer and fasting (1 Corinthians 7:4-6). Since fasting is typically not done for more than forty days at a time, couples who have abstained for months at a time are not taking into consideration God's full plan for their marriage.

If this sounds familiar and you aren't talking about your sex life, how do you start the conversation? How about starting now? This devotion gives you the opportunity to have some open conversation about the importance of sexual intimacy. Make a commitment to listen without becoming defensive or hurt. At the same time, the goal is to improve your marriage, not to tear down the other person.

Questions:

1. Have you ever considered that sexual intimacy is an important aspect of God's plan for your marriage?
2. Is each of you satisfied with the frequency of your sexual encounters?
3. What are some of the blessings that have come from good sexual intimacy?
4. Are there past hurts from your love life that seem hard or hurtful to talk about?

If you have hurt one another by diminishing the importance of intimacy in your relationship, take the opportunity to confess, forgive each other, and commit to improving this part of your marriage.

3.

Don't Miss Out!

I recently took care of a couple who had been together for more than twenty years. Sex had always been painful, but wasn't even possible for the last fifteen years. I think I have a lot of professional experience in the area of sexual dysfunction, but fifteen years is a long time to go without having sex! I warned the couple we were treading on difficult ground. I was careful to say that this issue didn't get to that point overnight, and that it was probably going to take us a while to make appreciable progress.

Then I examined the woman, and I knew we were in trouble. She had significant vaginal atrophy (a condition where the vagina is very dry and can shrink—she was over the age of 65) and could not tolerate even the smallest inserted instrument. I smiled, asked her to get dressed, and left the room. Standing in front of my computer, I asked for wisdom as I typed out a plan for the first four weeks of our journey together.

Now that was an extreme case, but not an isolated one. My speaking engagements have brought people into my office who tell me, "We had given up hope until we heard you speak." Although that may sound very flattering to most physicians, I frankly find it terrifying. I take my role as a physician very seriously – I want to help people, especially in the area of sexual dysfunction. Of course, I wish they would come to me in the first month of difficulty instead of the fifteenth year of problems! Many of these issues stem from a lack of communication that leads to despair.

Whether you are in your first week of marriage or have shared your bed for thirty years, you can always learn something about communicating with your lover. So if you think, as we do, that marriage is a journey and not a destination, buckle in and prepare to speak your mind! Oh, and the title of this chapter is dedicated to that couple I described. After nine weeks of therapy, medications, and communication, they were able to have sex without pain for the first time in fifteen years! Their response, obviously, was pure joy. They said, "We have been missing out!" The take-home message is this: Where there is love, there is always hope for a better encounter.

Questions:

1. Do you feel comfortable telling your spouse what feels good when you are being intimate?
2. How important is a fulfilling sex life in your marriage? If your answers are not the same, talk about other areas that you have had differences of opinion (parenting, finances, in-laws, etc.) and how you have resolved those differences.
3. What is your ideal for your sex life? This question could be answered in terms of sexual frequency, a partner experiencing climax, or a degree of openness.

4.

It's all About Priorities

I t is our hope that you have a satisfying sex life, and that your moments of intimacy are cherished for both quality and quantity. However, based on what we have seen in couples we work with, that may not be the case. Another question we have to ask is, "Have you made sex a priority?"

Many of my patients say that they come home, take care of the kids, put them to bed, and then start their own lengthy to-do list. At the end of all this, they collapse from exhaustion and fall asleep. When I inquire about what the husband is doing during this time, I get the typical response that he has his own things to do. In addition, he is usually up much later into the night. Many couples rarely go to bed at the same time. These conversations usually come up while I am addressing a complaint from a patient involving low sex drive. When I try to determine the cause, the patient and I quickly realize that even if there was a sexual desire, there is no time for sex. One of the suggestions I usually make is that they do their usual routine of putting the kids to bed, then consider some intimate time *before* the to-do list. I don't know too many husbands who will say no to sex because they have too many things to get done.

Many women report back that this plan works well. I've often wondered if the husband was truly busy or if he was dealing with a sense of rejection from his wife. In other words, the husband was probably trying to find something to do in order not to dwell on his feelings of frustration or disappointment.

For women, sex is kind of like exercise – if you get into the habit and it becomes part of your routine, you not only enjoy it more, but miss it when you don't have it. The best place to start is sometimes to plan out ahead of time when sexual encounters can occur during the week. This may seem to be a turn-off, but you have to start somewhere. Besides, planned sex is better than no sex! Think about it. You plan meals, shopping, kids' activities, work, church, etc. If you truly want to make sex a priority in your life, perhaps it's time to pencil in some time. Planned sex also does not have to be a chore. Just as you can plan an extravagant meal or a tasty burger and fries, you can plan to enjoy sex of any flavor!

Make a plan. Evaluate your next week together and decide which day (or days!) would be the best for intimacy.

Questions:

1. Are there other priorities or activities that routinely inter-fere with time for intimacy? (Examples could include cleaning the house after the kids go to bed, staying up late to watch TV, or finishing work from the office.)
2. Has past rejection caused either you or your spouse to fill up your evenings such that there is "no time" for sex?
3. Have you ever considered purposefully setting aside time for sex?
4. Are you willing to make time?

5.

Initiation: The Stand-Off

I'm often surprised when my patients have little intimate contact, but believe that their husbands are okay with that. With a few exceptions, such as medical conditions, many men have an ever-present sex drive. In a situation like this, the men often feel as if they have tried everything, but it hasn't worked. In order to avoid anger, or to prevent emotionally hurting their wives over this issue, they have often given up. That can lead to an even worse situation – saying that sexual abstinence is "okay." The very real threat is that this situation can make the man vulnerable to finding sexual fulfillment from other sources.

There are no excuses for stepping outside of your marriage for sexual fulfillment, but sexual droughts in a marriage can often create an environment where spouses make selfish choices.

There is temptation at every turn – pornography, co-workers, etc. While women may not desire sex, they do have a need for intimacy. The women can, therefore, become vulnerable to finding others to fulfill that need for connectedness.

Even if neither one has given in to other temptations, the couple is now in the situation where neither side is interested in initiating sexual encounters. Typically, the woman wants the man to show interest and to initiate the encounter. The man, however, is not interested in opening himself up again for rejection or an emotional outburst from the woman he loves. It is important to remember that men have an innate longing to be desired. They want to know that their wives want to have sex with them. Sometimes this is a quiet struggle; sometimes it can be more animated. Perhaps one or the other is confiding in friends rather than discussing the issue with each other. Whatever form it takes, it is a serious problem.

This is not a battle to be won or lost – both sides have already lost. Rather, it is a crisis in your marriage that needs to be solved together. As with most issues in marriage, a candid conversation can go a long way to address these problems.

If some breach of trust has led to this situation, additional help such as professional counseling may be needed and to determine what path should be taken.

Questions:

1. Are we at a standoff, waiting to see who will initiate?
2. What hurts keep each of us from initiating (both for the man and the woman)?
3. What habits do we have that keep us from starting intimate encounters?

6.

Painful Intercourse, part 1 - Physical Issues

W omen share the complaint of "painful intercourse" in one of two scenarios. Either they have a physical or medical reason for pain, or they have an emotional origin for the discomfort. Each of these scenarios requires a different approach, so in this chapter we will address the first scenario.

Many women have visited the gynecologist a month or two after the honeymoon, realizing they cannot have intercourse without pain. When there is pain when intercourse is even attempted, it is possible that there is some vaginal issue that needs to be addressed. Some women have a band of tissue called the hymen that is causing discomfort. This is most often addressed either with a minor surgical procedure to correct the problem or with an in-office procedure, depending on how much needs to be done. Women should consider these options if they have pain with (or inability to use) tampons or pap smears.

Infections can also cause pain. If either of you has had previous sexual partners, it is important that you have testing done to make sure that sexually transmitted infections (STIs) are not present. Some infections have no symptoms that bother patients except when they try to have sex. There are also infections that are not considered an STI that can cause discomfort. Testing for infection is an important part of the medical exam for determining the cause of painful intercourse.

Another consideration is, for lack of a better term, "nerve pain." This could be due to a vaginal delivery or other trauma. Some women have also experienced a back injury and will feel pain in the pelvis or vagina because the nerves to these parts start in the back. If you see a doctor and the exam is normal, you may want to talk to him or her about seeing a physical therapist who specializes in female issues like pelvic pain. There are many treatments for muscular or nerve pain, but not all doctors specialize in sexual dysfunction, so do not be afraid to ask detailed questions or to be referred to someone who treats the kind of pain you are having.

There are times when a lack of lubrication can be part of the problem. This is common in women who are breast feeding, women who have had a hysterectomy, and women who are going through menopause. If you are in one of these situations, consider trying a good lubricant. I often tell women that vaginal dryness is similar to dry skin on other parts of the body. If your hands are dry and flaky, you would use a lotion. You may already know that you have vaginal dryness, or you may need an exam to determine that this is a problem for you. However, take care to avoid irritants. Some women do fine with over-the-counter lubricants; other women use something more natural like organic coconut oil. Oil and silicon-based lubricants last longer, but may cause more irritation than water-based lubricants. Finding the best product for you may take some experimentation.

The basic point of this chapter is that pain with intercourse is common and treatable. It is not normal for sex to hurt, so seek medical treatment if this is a problem for you.

Questions:

1. Have you had discomfort during intercourse that you have been unwilling to address?
2. After reading this section, do any of these scenarios describe the discomfort you are experiencing?
3. Are you willing to seek professional help to diagnose and treat the source of your pain?

7.

Painful Intercourse, part 2 – Emotional Concerns

Physical issues are not always the blame when patients complain of painful intercourse. Another common cause of pain with intercourse is the inability to relax. Many women have been raised to believe sex is taboo and dirty, then they get married and sex is suddenly supposed to be this great experience they share with their husbands. The problem is that sometimes the brain cannot make that quick switch. What starts as honeymoon shyness can turn into an inability to form an intimate connection. Many times men begin to take this personally. They can become frustrated as time goes on and become unable to figure out a way to approach their wives in the bedroom.

Another consideration is that some women do not feel comfortable in their own skin. Allowing their partner to see them naked makes them cringe. I have taken care of patients who have been married for a decade or more and their spouses have never seen them without their clothes on. There could be a history of hurtful comments that have caused one or both partners to feel self-conscious and unwilling to expose themselves. If your bodies belong to one another, yet the lights are always off or you change in separate rooms to avoid your spouse seeing your body, you may need to seek professional counseling to help you work on your intimate life.

If you are uncomfortable with your body, relaxing during a sexual experience will be nearly impossible, ensuring that sex will be uncomfortable or even painful. Orgasm is not possible under these circumstances. Sometimes this leads couples to think that experiencing orgasm is not God's plan for them. Reassurance from your spouse can help restore confidence in your relationship, but you may also need to seek professional help to move forward.

Compounding this issue, sometimes men are insensitive and say or do things that strike a nerve or instantly shut their wives down. This can lead to a breach in communication and more hurt feelings. Because God made men and women to be different, women can be easily offended, and men can be easily frustrated about the lack of sex that can result from the offenses. Sometimes, being willing to take the first step toward reconciliation, even if you do not feel you are the cause of the rift, can lead to healing and improved closeness.

Simply discussing your background and base of knowledge about sex may improve things. You may, however, need to seek professional help to work through the barriers to intimacy.

Questions:

1. How was sex viewed by your family of origin? Was it taboo or never discussed or was there communication about God's plan for sex?

2. Are you comfortable with your partner seeing you naked? What makes you uncomfortable? How can you work together to change the situation? Be creative and try to create a plan on which you can both agree.

8.

Lack of Orgasm in Women – Medical Considerations

I saw a patient the other day who had been married for almost two decades. She was new to my office, so I began my usual list of questions: Do you have pain with sex? Are you able to orgasm? She looked at me curiously and said, "Why do you ask?" I explained to her that I treat sexual dysfunction and find that many women will only tell me about a problem if I ask a direct question. She went on to tell me she had never had an orgasm and had decided there was something wrong with her.

Many women I see have never had an orgasm. Sometimes it is simply a lack of education about female anatomy and where the nerves are that evoke sensual pleasure; this is something that the couple (not just the woman) needs to explore. There are many good books written by Christians for Christians that explain the semantics of sexual enjoyment. If there is still a lack of orgasm after reviewing some good material, I recommend an exam and discussion with a gynecologist. If there are no medical concerns, a consultation with a sex therapist is helpful to allow couples to explore ways to improve this part of their sex lives.

Sometimes, as briefly touched on in the previous chapter, women are unable to relax enough to experience climax. This is typically more common early in marriage, as everything is new and women have been told to stay covered and protect themselves from premarital sex, but then they often have trouble transitioning to allowing their spouse to explore their body. A little shyness is normal, but a consistent inability to relax during intimacy can become a big problem. Couples can continue to communicate and work through this, often with the help of a close mentor or therapist.

There are also times that dishonesty has existed in the couples' sex life. What I mean by this is that women have often "faked it." Faking an orgasm seems an easy way out for some women. Since many men take less time to climax than women, it is a quick way to be done with the encounter. The problem with this cycle is that the husband thinks he has figured out how to pleasure his wife and thus repeats the pattern. The wife then has to either continue to fake it or come clean and tell him what he is doing doesn't work for her. Although there are times that something feels good one day but not the next, you will never have a fulfilling sex life without honest communication.

Sometimes, men have decided that pleasuring their wives is not a necessary part of intercourse. They achieve climax, roll over and go to sleep. This may have started as a lack of communication that evolved into his resignation that things won't change. Women may have given up experiencing sexual intimacy and pleasure either because communication hasn't worked in the past, because they want to "get it over with," or because of a variety of other reasons. This may lead to decreased frequency of sex and frustration on the part of both partners.

Questions:

1. Has there been a pattern of unsatisfying sexual encounters in your relationship? If your answers are not the same, discuss the difference in your satisfaction with sexual encounters.

2. What is one thing you do that you think your spouse enjoys? Be honest about how much you like (or don't like) the other person's answer.

3. What is one thing you would like your spouse to do during sex? If the answer makes you uncomfortable, discuss why and be open and honest about your discomfort.

9.

Our own Private Playground—
What is and is not "Off-Limits"

This short chapter is full of risk. It is full of liberty, and anytime you have liberty, you have the opportunity to misuse that liberty. I have no desire to impose my discomforts or comforts upon you. However, sticking our heads in the sand and pretending there are no questions about what is and is not okay to bring in the bedroom is a very dangerous ignorance to embrace. Rather, we should experience the freedom found in being able to discuss what is and is not welcome in our lives involving sexual issues. Just like a discussion about any other liberty, it is first important to understand that God has boundaries of safety set up to protect us from the broken nature of our hearts.

Enter into the grown-up playground of your love life! This is an amazing playground that may include sex toys and equipment made just for you and your spouse. Endless opportunity for pleasure abounds, but watch out! There are also toys and equipment that lie just outside of the fence, maybe even in another couples' playground, that were not designed for you or your spouse. You have the blessing of playing with anything that is within your boundaries. You also have the responsibility of playing with the equipment the way it was intended. Understand that you are not required to use anything on the playground. God has given you the freedom to choose, but He has also given you a responsibility to honor the boundaries He has in place.

So ask yourself and your spouse, "Why do we want to use a specific item?" Only you will know the true intentions of your heart. Here are some of the boundaries God has in place for all playgrounds.

1. This playground is for the two of you only! No third parties involved in thought or deed.
2. Anything that demeans or belittles you or your spouse is *not allowed*.
3. No hurting of each other is allowed physically, emotionally, or spiritually.
4. If the toy or activity becomes the focus/priority, you must leave it behind.
5. Both of you must agree to what is used.

Within those boundaries, you have so much freedom.

Some things are like a good, old-fashioned swing set. They are gentle and provide reliable, long-lasting pleasure. They are fairly safe. Other items may seem like the most absurd rollercoaster ride you could *never* imagine. These may entail a bit more risk. Either way, as you enter into this playground you and your beloved are probably going to have some items on which you don't agree. Instead of focusing on what you don't agree on, look at what you both would like to enjoy.

The whole idea of adding a prop to your intimate times should be about adding to your level of fun and intimacy. This tends to be a touchy subject, especially in Christian circles. In truth, many times the desire to bring toys into the bedroom comes from what has been seen in pornography and many of the toys out there are produced by the porn industry. Who you are supporting with your purchase should be a consideration.

Questions:

1. What are some of your fears as you start to talk about this subject?
2. What areas of the playground are you curious about?
3. Are there any specific items that you do not feel comfortable with?

10.

Experimentation in the Bedroom

W ith all this talk of what you do and do not want to add to your love life, it is important to briefly touch upon how to implement some new ideas. There is no way to cover all of the possible ways that appeal to couples, so we will stick with some good principles to live by.

Principle #1- Keep to the stuff that is beneficial and don't make stuff the focus.

A wise man named Paul once said "Everything is permissible for me - but not everything is beneficial. Everything is permissible for me" - but I will not be mastered by anything," (1 Cor. 6:12, NIV 1984).

I think that it would be a fair application of this passage to say, while you have a great amount of freedom in what you do in the bedroom, do not allow yourself or your spouse to be so focused on the new and exciting adventure that the new item, position, or roles you play become the focus.

Later, Paul reiterates the same language with a different twist on the end. "You say, 'I am allowed to do anything,' but not everything is good for you. You say, 'I am allowed to do anything,' but not everything is beneficial. Don't be concerned for your own good but for the good of others," (1 Cor. 10:23-24, NLT).

This new twist identifies that the most important point we should consider is not the freedoms that we have, but rather the responsibility we have to our spouses to consider them first.

Principle #2 - Have Fun!

In therapy, I am always looking for ways to incorporate humor. A good sense of humor and the ability to laugh at stuff that is funny are important in helping people get past difficult obstacles. It is important that a person also pays attention to timing and sensitivities. For example, it is *never* okay to ignore the feedback you are getting from your audience. If your spouse is not laughing or enjoying your humor, *it is not fun or funny*! A light heart of exploration and enjoyment is the key to an enjoyable time.

Principle #3 - Don't lose sight of why you are there!

All the experimentation in the world cannot compensate for two people who don't want to love each other completely or for a bad lover. Both of you must be taking your adventures in lovemaking for the purpose of furthering your enjoyment, not compensating for an unhappy relationship. You are there to enjoy each other and to share in an amazing pleasure only given to married couples. Whatever you do, don't fight about experimenting.

Principle #4 - Get help when you are stuck.

Shameless plug: If you have struggles with orgasm or physical limitations, get help. A well-trained sex therapist and/or ob/gyn can help with most issues. Be sure that you align with them theologically. Start by asking them, "What is your theology of sex?" If they are not willing to discuss how they believe God views sex or if they say, "Anything goes," you should probably see a red flag. Sometimes sexual issues are complex and sometimes they are easy, but either way it may be hard to see the answers when you are stuck in the middle.

Questions:

1. Have there been times when you felt like you were trying too hard to "do something different" and lost sight of just enjoying making love?

2. What are ways that you could make one another feel more comfortable to try new things?

3. Do you think there are any areas where you are stuck without a solution and should get some help?

11.

Past Hurts and Redefining Your Sex Life

If you come into your marriage with no previous exposure to sex and have not engaged in intense sexual activity with your spouse until you were married, consider yourself very blessed. For the rest of us, we must deal with past hurts, guilt, trauma, or abuse that has warped our understanding of healthy sexuality. That understanding can also be marred by unhealthy messages about sex given unintentionally from our parents or mentors. In dealing with a world that is sex saturated and where abuse and exposure are rampant, many (if not most) couples come together with a litany of past sexual hurts. It is imperative to seek forgiveness and healing from these hurts so you may experience the fullness of true sexual unity.

Healthy guilt frequently comes into play when we have pursued a physical relationship prematurely, looked at pornography or fantasized about someone. This guilt should be dealt with by seeking forgiveness and turning away from the behavior. It is at this point that guilt should subside. On the other hand, if you have already sought forgiveness from God and have repented, any remaining guilt is not from God but rather from Satan. Don't let him steal your happiness by allowing him to tear you down again.

Unhealthy guilt is found when you have sought forgiveness but continue in guilt or when you are a victim of sexual abuse or exposure. Frequently, rape victims will experience guilt for what was done to them when clearly the blame belongs to the rapist. Guilt for sexual dreams is also common but unwarranted.

This book is not a replacement for therapy. If you are working on how to deal with exposure to porn and/or past relationships that have been too physical, you may be able to start that process of healing right here. Deeper sexual trauma is addressed in the next chapter.

Redefining your sex life needs to start with resolving issues from the past so you can move forward toward a healthy relationship. Make sure that as you approach this subject with each other that grace and humility are primary in your discussion.

Questions:

1. Are there any unhealthy or weird messages that your parents gave you about sex or sexuality?
2. Are there times when you feel guilty about past experiences or exposures? If so, stop and pray now for God to begin that healing process.
3. Are there aspects of your marital sex life that you feel guilty about?

12.

History of Sexual Trauma

We live in a fallen world. Men take advantage of women, women manipulate men with sex, adults harm children, and people step out of the bounds of marriage to serve their own evil, selfish desires. Sometimes, men or women have been sexually abused and then find it difficult to move forward with intimacy in their marriage. If you have experienced sexual trauma but have not sought out the help of a professional counselor or therapist, we encourage you to take that first step toward healing.

If your partner has experienced sexual trauma, it can be very difficult to move forward with your intimate life. You may say or do things that unknowingly trigger painful memories, causing your spouse to shut down or reject sexual touch. This can leave you feeling frustrated or angry, especially if your spouse has difficulty articulating his or her feelings or is unwilling to talk about the events that are triggering the negative response.

If you are the one who has experienced trauma, I encourage you to communicate openly with your spouse. If you have identified the words or actions that cause you anxiety or flash backs, it is important that you voice your concerns to your spouse. Trained counselors can help you work through your feelings and help you and your spouse create new memories and new avenues of communication.

I have had some women say to me that they just want to be normal again. They tearfully say that the sexual abuse or rape changed them and made them distrust men. They want a "normal" sex life with their husbands, but simply don't know how to get there.

This one page chapter is simply not sufficient to heal past hurts and move you to a new place of intimacy. Simply being honest about your past and allowing your spouse into the traumatic parts of your past will bring you closer together. Explore together how you can move forward and support each other as you seek God's best for your intimate life.

Questions:

1. Has your spouse done something in the bedroom that triggered a painful memory? Share the specific thing that reminds you of a past hurt.

2. Do you have secrets about your past that you have been unwilling to share? Discuss if seeing a counselor would help you communicate your hurts and needs as you move forward.

13.

Foreplay

Foreplay can be divided into two major categories: priming and persuading. Priming pertains to the physical touch and caress that go into preparing your spouse for intercourse and/or orgasm. Persuading (think, "pursuit") is the physical, emotional, and spiritual effort that raises desire for intimacy in your spouse. This chapter will cover priming, and the next chapter will cover the aspect of persuading.

Sadly, so little is actually taught about the physical aspects of sex in Christian circles, and what is known is stumbled into or, worse, never realized. The best lovers in the world do not have to be experienced; they have to be intentional. Foreplay, in varying amounts, is essential to great lovemaking. The intention of foreplay generally differs between the genders. For women, foreplay allows the vagina to lubricate and extend internally and for the labia and the clitoris to engorge with blood, much like the penis. If foreplay does not happen, it is possible that the female could experience a large amount of pain rather than pleasure when intercourse occurs. Additionally, foreplay allows women to get their minds and emotions focused on enjoying sex. In men, foreplay allows for the penis to engorge and prepare for intercourse as well as allows for the opportunity for stronger or enhanced orgasms.

Yes, this sounds so very clinical. Essentially, foreplay gives us an opportunity to enjoy the pleasure of seeing our spouses receive pleasure.

In general, men will respond to friction by reaching orgasm. In many ways, it is a simple equation of erection, friction, and orgasm. Women are not designed to respond that way. Orgasm is only reached when her mind and body are headed in the same direction and when physical stimulation meets her needs at the time. Thus comes the never-ending conundrum for men: what worked yesterday may not work today! This is why communication is vital. Remember, sex is supposed to be fun!

Okay, so what about the "quickie"? There are times when both of you are in the mood, at the same time. If that is the case, there should not be any issues with "quickies." However, as you can probably imagine, that will not always be the case. If quick sexual encounters without foreplay become the basis of your sex life, you are also missing out on a deeper intimacy. The quality of your sex life will not be as good as it can (and should) be. Remember: all orgasms are great, but there are definitely some better than others!

Questions:

1. What physical foreplay do you like? What physical foreplay do you not like?
2. What things would you like your spouse to do that he or she doesn't currently do?
3. What things would you like your spouse to do more often?
4. Do you think it is ever okay to skip foreplay (the quickie question)?

14.

Non-Physical Foreplay

T his chapter covers the non-physical aspects of foreplay. Men, pay attention! Women have a tendency to need more of both physical and non-physical foreplay, and *both* are important. Certainly, men need non-physical foreplay as well. However, their need is frequently overridden by the presence of opportunities to be physically intimate.

Something as fantastic as sexual intercourse takes preparation and warrants savoring each course of the meal. Yet, this often causes confusion for males. Men tend to underestimate the need for non-physical stimulation. Remember, this aspect of foreplay is about persuasion and pursuit. For men, it can be difficult to understand why their spouses would not want to have sexual intercourse anytime and all of the time when it feels so good.

Step beyond the frustrating stereotypes. For those of you who do this part of your love life well, let this serve as a reminder to enjoy and indulge. For the other men, let it serve as an encouragement to do lovemaking well.

Persuasion is best found in loving well. By knowing the areas that speak volumes of love to your spouse, and then acting on that knowledge, you give an opportunity for feelings to arise. In the absence of that action, however, sexual desire will tend to drop significantly. For example, if you know your wife/husband especially appreciates a vacuumed floor (or homework done with the kids, a well-prepared meal, clean dishes, a balanced checkbook, etc.), then do these often! All of these actions impact the general atmosphere in the marriage.

Men, don't just attend church. Listen intently, sing joyfully, pray earnestly and implement these positive actions throughout the week. Your genuine worship will spark a flame in her. When you take on your God-intended role of spiritual leadership in your family, it makes your wife want to serve you and care for you. You become more attractive to her and, in turn, your pursuit of God causes you to treat her as Christ intended.

Be careful, though! Don't do things around the house looking at sex as being some kind of reward for good behavior. However, if the dishes are done, more time will be freed up! Non-physical foreplay really boils down to having the desire and undertaking the action in serving one another.

Questions:

1. Is there something that your spouse does or says that lets you know he or she would like to have sex that evening? Do you each have a signal?
2. What things can your spouse do or say that help you feel appreciated and open to pursuing sex?
3. Are there things that your spouse does or says that "kill the mood"?

15.

Pornography and its Effects, part 1: What Men and Women are Learning from Porn

---

People are tired of talking about porn. Unfortunately, they are not tired of looking at it. As a $13 billion/year industry, it is not slowing down. Pornography is being discussed here because it creates unrealistic expectations about sex and about your partner.

Here is what porn teaches men:

- Women are always in the mood for sex
- Women are automatically turned on by any touch
- Women are always orgasmic
- Having sex in different positions is imperative
- Women like to be dominated
- All women are vocal during sex

- The best sex partners look like they are between the ages of 18 and 24
- Sex is not about relationship, it is about aggressive pursuit
- Women are frequently having sex with other women
- Sex is just sex; it is not personal
- All women can and will have an orgasm through vaginal or anal sex

Porn teaches women:

- I have to be orgasmic (and often multiple times) to be normal
- I have to look like I am a 20-year-old with a perfect body to be desirable
- I should enjoy being dominated and frequently humiliated during sex
- I should be overwhelmed with pleasure, no matter where I am touched
- Having sex with other women (or multiple other people) is normal
- Men should be able to have sex for hours and not reach climax until they have exhausted every position and person in the room

Ultimately, porn writes a script for the way we should experience sex. Most of that script is full of unreasonable expectations. The script deadens the meaning of sex to being impersonal and meaningless other than with the sole goal of physical satisfaction.

It teaches us that finding someone who is sexually compatible is a matter of searching for that person rather than growing in your relationship. Porn says that sex should always be our goal in our relationship and always be available. It says there is something wrong with you if you don't want sex. Ultimately, it is an easy way to invite a virtual 3rd, 4th, 5th etc. person into your relationship without taking any risk of STD's or pregnancy. However, you do get infected with the cancer of dissatisfaction, un-real expectations, and dysfunctional desire that return worse than nagging mosquitoes in Minnesota. When a person is looking at porn there is a subtle but sure erosion of the bond between, and the exclusivity of, a marital sex life.

You may be getting the idea that I do not think porn is healthy. Exactly. Porn is also instinctively linked with masturbation. Please read about that in a later chapter.

Questions:

1. What defenses have you built to protect your family from purposeful or accidental porn exposure?
2. What kinds of emotions do you experience when you consider that your spouse has been exposed to pornography?
3. What are some ways you can help repair the damage from previous exposure to pornography?

16.

Pornography and its Effects, part 2: When Porn Becomes the Solution for Lack of Intimacy

So we have made our case for why porn is not healthy for individuals and couples, but what happens when it has already invaded and done its damage? What happens when it is invited into the relationship? Or, perhaps it is allowed just because sex is not going well. Maybe one of you does not have a desire to have sex, so it is permitted for the other to partake. Have you heard yourself say, "His drive is so strong that I can't or don't want to keep up, so at least he isn't cheating," or, "Maybe we can fire up our love life by watching a little bit"? On the other hand, what if someone is turning to pornography as a perceived solution to some other dysfunction in your sexual relationship?

No matter the reason, the hard truth is that porn creates a chasm between husband and wife. For the purposes of this discussion, it's not just explicit pornography that is at issue – it can be provocative movies, shows, or even books.

This is a perspective issue. You may or may not currently agree with this position. However, this is my experience with couples over the past decade.

Porn reaches into the human psyche. It accelerates and heightens desires that cannot be quenched in or out of the marriage because it draws a picture of a physical relationship that cannot be replicated in real life. It is a fantasy world with great editing. You only get to see the orgasm, not the fallout. Another issue is that it will always leave the viewer longing for more. Most of the time, something with more intensity or something new is desired with each viewing. It is a pursuit of the same level of "enjoyment."

The intent may be to improve a sexual dysfunction with the use of porn, but the reality is that it leaves all parties feeling alone, distant, used, guilty and dissatisfied. Rather than an aid to your sexual relationship, it will only create deeper issues. It is no substitute for the intimacy that you should be experiencing in your own sexual relationship! One of the reasons for this book is our desire that you and your spouse cultivate a healthy and rewarding sex life. Porn is not a solution!

If the use of pornography is more deeply rooted than simple casual use or shared use with your spouse, then there may be addiction involved. For these cases, we recommend seeking additional help or counseling to overcome this barrier in your sexual relationship.

Questions:

1. Has there ever been a tacit, or even explicit approval of the use of pornography in your relationship?
2. If porn is somehow involved in your relationship, what is the underlying reason? Are there other ways to meet those needs?
3. How can you support your spouse in an effort to rid your relationship of porn?

17.

Masturbation: The Third Rail of Sex Discussions

First, as is on all the subjects we have discussed, we can always agree to disagree. Don't tune out truth in one area just because you disagree in another. I am prone to being wrong, just like all humans.

There are no scripture verses that speak specifically about masturbation, so that leaves us to draw conclusions based on how our discussion otherwise aligns with the Word of God. With masturbation, we can make informed decisions on the subject based upon the circumstances under which it happens and the physical and mental impact of the activity. It is difficult and dangerous to speak on issues where God is silent. We should, therefore, walk through this topic with grace and humility.

I believe that it is possible for masturbation to occur without sinning. It is not, however, very probable. Masturbation is physical stimulation of erogenous or "feel-good" zones for the purpose of sexual satisfaction outside of intercourse. In men, it is almost always done with objective of reaching orgasm. In women, orgasm is frequently, but not always, the objective. Touching your own body is not a sin. Orgasms are not sinful. The problem really stems from what is going on in the mind. Masturbation is rarely separate from fantasy. Who is the object of that fantasy? If it is your spouse, are you simply objectifying him or her? If it is someone else, didn't Christ himself say that was adultery?

For most men that I have worked with, the objective for masturbation has been reaching release as quickly as possible. This is not good training for being a good lover. There is not really an argument to be made for knowing your body and what feels good either, since orgasms in men are fairly easily achieved through stimulation of the penis. At the same time, I am not talking about special circumstances such as medical impediments or long-term separation for a job or military service.

For women that I have worked with, the objective has been to either satisfy a sexual release that their husbands were not willing or don't know how to provide, or to better know their own body. Women, having a much more complex road to orgasm (in that it is not simply a matter of friction on the clitoris), may have more leeway here. There may be a case to be made for self-exploration for the sake of understanding what feels good. There may also be a reasonable argument to be made for allowing engaged women to pursue some use of dilators or their hands in order to prepare themselves for marriage.

For either gender, a primary question that I would ask is: "Is your pursuit of masturbation really just unwillingness to show self-control?" Most people have surges of sexual desire and longing at times when their spouse is not available. That is a biological reality. I believe, however, that we are called daily to *be beyond our biology*. We cannot simply allow our hearts and minds to be slaves to our hormones.

So...If the mind can be clear of lust and objectification, if it is not secretly done (meaning that both husband and wife are aware and agree) and we are not placing ourselves as slave to our urges, there may be room for masturbation.

Depending on where you stand on masturbation, this can be a difficult topic to discuss. My intent is to not place you or your spouse in a situation of having to be deceitful or uncomfortable about this subject. Rather, please use this time to evaluate (if necessary) your actions and thoughts on this topic.

Questions:

1. Have you ever thought about God's heart regarding masturbation? What conclusions did you come to?
2. What (if anything) were you ever taught about masturbation and its permissiveness?
3. Based on what you know now, do you believe that masturbation is honoring to your spouse?
4. What is the most uncomfortable aspect of this topic to discuss?

18.

Praying Together

Do you feel comfortable praying out loud? Have you ever heard someone pray to God like they were talking to a close friend and marveled at their ability to communicate with his creator? It is certainly true that we have many different views of prayer. When a man and woman pray together, it can be one of the most intimate experiences in life. I tell teenaged girls and single women to avoid praying by themselves with a man as it can lead to...well, other things.

The Bible puts it this way, "Confess your sins to each other and pray for each other so that you may be healed. The earnest prayer of a righteous person has great power and produces wonderful results," (James 5:16, NLT). In this book, we have asked you to do some dangerous and scary things in order to accomplish sexual healing in your marriage. Prayer cannot be left off the list of things you must do to achieve complete healing. If you have not made prayer a part of your married life thus far, here are a few tips for how to get started.

Talk to God like you are talking to a friend. Ask your spouse how you can pray for him – what things are a struggle right now? How does she feel about work or raising the kids or her relationships with family and friends? Keep a running list of specific requests. Consider keeping a prayer journal together where you list prayer requests and when God shows you the answer, write it down. This can serve two purposes. The first is there are times that you may struggle with communication and having a list of things you are seeking God for as a couple can help draw you together again. As God answers prayers, seeing how He has worked in your lives is a faith builder. When things are difficult, you can remind each other of God's goodness and answers to your prayers.

I am not a big fan of scripted prayers, but there are times that they help us to say what has been on our hearts but we have difficulty articulating. After you answer the questions, consider praying the prayer out loud together. We suggest you pray together every night if possible, or as often as your schedules allow. Pray without ceasing for your spouse, your marriage, and your family and you will see God move mountains in your life.

Dear God,

We thank you for giving us each other. We confess that we need you to help us communicate and love each other as you intended. We want to honor you with our lives and serve you together. Please help us to grow more intimate and meet each other's sexual needs and desires. Protect us from hurt as we explore things that are scary and uncomfortable. Help us to seek you first in all we do and make us a living testimony of your power to change lives. In the name of Jesus we pray, amen.

Questions:

1. Have you made it a habit to pray together? If not, what keeps you from praying together? If so, have you made your spouse's needs the subject of your prayers?

2. James 4:3 tells us that we ask but do not receive - What do you need God to do in your marriage – perform a miracle, or just help you improve on a wonderful relationship?

3. Make a list together of specific requests for you as individuals, and in your marriage as a whole. Pick one or two things each night to pray for, out loud and together, asking God to strengthen your bond to each other and to Him.

19.

I'm a Good Lover, Right?

So, how do you know if you are a good lover? I suppose a good place to start would be to ask the object of your love (your spouse). There are times that you may be the unselfish lover – patient, kind, pursuing pleasure for your spouse. There may also be times that you are tired, insensitive, or just frustrated in general and loving becomes more sex and less intimacy.

If you have had prolonged periods of separation, either living in separate places or just not connecting physically, when you try to resume sex it can be very difficult. During this time of reconnecting, it is more important than ever to make the effort to be a good lover. So what are some qualities of a good lover?

-Puts the needs and desires of his partner above his own.

-Takes the time to understand what her partner enjoys during intimacy and makes the effort to do those things well.

-Asks questions when he is not certain about a new experience – toy, position, etc.—and listens even when his lover's answer is not what he would like.

-Yields to her lover's desire for intimacy at times when she would rather be selfish and not have sex.

-Works through times of difficulty in his marriage, responding with love and tenderness in order to protect his spouse from temptation.

This is just the short list, but you get the idea. There are times that you (and I, for that matter!) have been great lovers. We have been kind and patient, loving our spouses and expressing that love through physical touch. There are also times, however, that we have not been good lovers. We have rejected our spouses when we didn't "feel like it." We have gone for the quickie because we had other things to do, when our spouses were longing for more of our time and attention.

When some aspect of your marriage has been anything but great, how do you change? The same way you change anything else in life – through genuine repentance and work toward restoration. Remember, intimacy in marriage takes two people. Though a major rift may have started with the actions or emotions of one spouse, that rift is often widened by the hurt and anger of the other spouse.

We serve a great God who promises to heal and restore. We need only ask for forgiveness from Him and our lover and commit to renewing our passion for one another.

Questions:

1. Has there been a time (or period of time) that you know you have been a selfish lover? What steps can you take to improve intimacy?

2. Have you failed to teach your spouse how to pleasure you? What emotions have held you back in pursuit of good loving (fear of rejection, anxiety of being judged, etc.)?

3. Confess to your spouse your anger or hurt over the past, and express forgiveness. If the hurts run too deep for a simple "sorry," commit to seeking professional help together.

20.

How Often Should We Do It?

"How often should we do it?" "What is "normal"?" Have you ever asked those questions? Frequency is an enduring topic. It seems to come up in every marriage at some point. Sex ignites very powerful emotions in us when we have it and when we do not. It is no wonder that many couples spend lots of time embattled over the subject. Whether you realize it or not, you may be sending a blitz of messages to your spouse in the midst of differing desires.

If his desire is higher than hers, she may be receiving messages like:

- He thinks of nothing but sex.
- All he wants me for is sex.
- He is never satisfied.
- If I give him more, he will just want more.

Meanwhile, he may be thinking:

- She hates sex.
- She never wants sex.
- She does not care about my needs.

On the other hand, if her desire is higher than his, she may be thinking:

- There is something wrong with me.
- I am not attractive to him
- He must be getting his needs met somewhere else.

He may be thinking:

- This rocks!

Here is a frequent hiccup especially found when a husband's desire is higher than his wife's. She worries that he will never be satisfied and will always want more, so she withholds out of fear that she will just make the "problem" grow if she offers to have sex more. In truth, most couples that I have worked with find that as she starts to have sex with him more, he becomes satisfied with much less than what he (or she) thought he wanted. It should be noted that the great feeling of having your wife long to be intimate with you results in a temporary surge of desire (no more than three million times a day for the first month or so). Throwing out numbers is not going to be helpful, but setting realistic expectations will be. Healthy frequency is found when a husband and wife mutually seek to serve each other.

Questions:

1. It's time to have the discussion about frequency. Are you having sex as much as each of you desires?
2. How often do you desire to have sex?
3. What do you think is "normal"?
4. If your expectations are not the same, can you commit to work with each other to resolve these differences?

21.

We're Different – When He Has a Lower Sex Drive than She Does

———❦———

The discouragement that comes from feeling like you and your struggles are different from all of those around you can be paralyzing. Often when wives have a higher drive or desire for sex than their husbands, there is a huge amount of self-talk that is unhealthy. A few of these destructive thoughts are:

1.   I must be some kind of slut or sex addict.

It follows the social phenomenon that when guys sleep around in high school or college they are thought of as studs, but girls who sleep around are sluts. Women will often believe that there must be something wrong with them if they enjoy sex and want to have it frequently.

2.   He is getting his needs met elsewhere.

Along the same lines, the belief remains that *all* guys want sex *all* the time. If my husband is not taking advantage of my high libido, then he must be either masturbating all the time or having an affair.

3. My husband doesn't find me attractive anymore.

With all of the beautiful women out there, he must be losing interest in me. After all, I am not eighteen anymore. I have put on some weight, my breasts aren't as perky and well...I have just lost it.

4. He must be gay.

I wondered why he wanted to go hang out with the guys more than stay home with me. He has been really good about sitting down and watching chick-flicks.

You get the point. As much as these ideas are tongue in cheek, the thoughts really plague some women. While I can't specifically say that these thoughts are always wrong, I would recommend that you start with trying to adjust your perspective.

First, recognize that God intended for us to completely enjoy and desire sex. You may be blessed with a body that is fantastically responsive. Your husband may need an award for being a great lover and making sure that your pleasure is so intense you can't seem to get enough. Or you may naturally have a high libido due to higher testosterone levels. Any way you slice it, enjoying and wanting sex is good.

Secondly, work hard at not putting your husband in a box. Not all men have high libidos. Most men experience changes in their desire as they go through different life stages. In many ways, guys have been socially trained to believe that they must have a high sex drive when in reality if they are living without pornography and all kinds of sexual stimuli outside of the marriage, their libidos may come down quite a bit. When that drive is less, then things might be going well. Many other issues can account for lowered sex drive, to include lower testosterone levels, health problems, children (just like women) or just a change in their perspective that tells them your relationship is so much more than just sex.

Third. Big reality check time. Most women depicted in pornography are depicted to look between the ages of 18-26. You will only fit in that age group for eight years max. After that you will age. *That is okay!* You do not need to look like you are twenty-six for the rest of your life. God could have kept us all looking that age if he wanted to. Marital love transcends external appearance. That is not a pass on looking nice for your spouse or taking care of your body; it is a reminder that we all age. Having persistent joy allows us to look and feel young regardless of our age.

Lastly, many couples struggle with mismatched levels of desire. If your husband (or wife for that matter) has lower desire than you, it does not mean that he is homosexual. As we have stated, many things could be at play. If there is a struggle with same-sex attraction, it is time to get therapeutic help, but don't just jump to that conclusion.

This may sound crazy, but usually his answers to a lower sex drive are just as reasonable as hers. If answers to the following questions are tough to say or find, ask for help by sitting down with a trusted therapist.

Questions:

1. Ask your wife what she thinks about why your libido is lower.
2. Discuss what reasons you think are driving the discrepancy.
3. What would be a good frequency for sex that the two of you could work toward?

22.

His Need to be Desired by His Wife

I t is well known that women have a need to be cared for and to be loved by their husbands. It is common to talk about men as being sensitive if they know how to comfort their wives, or if they cry when she cries, etc. What is often overlooked is that a man needs to know that his wife desires him. Not just that she desires sex or desires intimacy, but that she actually wants *him*.

Men and women face many pressures. Men, traditionally speaking, feel pressured to work hard and be the best at the office or on the court or pretty much anywhere. When they do not feel like their wife is "in their corner," they may begin looking elsewhere for affirmation. This seemingly innocent pursuit of affirmation can be the start to an emotional or physical relationship outside their marriage.

How can women protect the men they love? Show your man that you desire him. Hug and kiss him frequently. Tell him he is physically attractive to you, that you are excited about him coming home. Send him a text or email during the day just to remind him that you love him and are thinking about him. When you love on and show desire to your husband, you protect him emotionally and help decrease his struggles with sexual temptation.

Men want to have sex with their wives. They also want their wives to *want* to have sex with them. It is this desire that leads to the greatest intimacy between two people.

So, if this open display of desire for your husband has not been part of your married life, where do you start? Here are some suggestions, followed by questions to help open the lines of communication between you and your spouse.

- Hold hands, touch his leg, stroke his hair. My grandma always said that recliners had no place in the living room of married people. She was on to something! If you are in recliners, you are not touching! Sit close and engage in non-sexual touch.
- Hug and kiss him hello and good bye. This may seem simple enough, but a physical connection a couple times a day will help you build a foundation for emotional connectedness.
- Leave him a note, send a text, or call in the middle of the day just to tell him you're thinking about him. This is especially important when you are working to rebuild intimacy in your marriage.
- Tell him he looks sexy. Tell him he has a nice...well, whatever you like about him. Not just once – tell him often

until he actually believes you are being sincere. This may seem awkward at first, but remember there are women out there that will happily tell your husband what they like about him, so protect him by making him secure in your eyes.

Questions:

1. Ask your husband if there are other things he would like you to do to express your love and desire for him. Admit to him if you are uncomfortable with a suggestion, but be open to trying new things.
2. Tell your husband if you have fears about opening up about your desires. Share your heart with him so he can understand where you are coming from.
3. Pray for each other – for emotional security, desire to make your married life stronger, and the ability to support one another in your need for intimacy.

23.

Creating the Environment – Protecting Your Spouse from Sexual Sin

———————————•———————————

In the culture that we live in, marriage is under attack. In many ways, it has become disposable. There are many factors that can cause a marriage to fail, such as financial, emotional or spiritual issues. Unfortunately, many couples ignore the sexual aspects of a healthy marriage. When it comes to finances, couples that have healthy interaction will spend hours talking about the future, budgeting, discussing major purchases, investments, day-to-day expenses and the like. When those things are not done, it inevitably leads a couple to argue about finances. In the extreme cases, disagreements about finances can lead to divorce. It should come as no surprise that couples that spend little time communicating about their sex life will struggle in this area as well.

If you want your finances to be safeguarded in your marriage, you make budgets and plans. You agree to do your best to work towards mutual future goals. In the same way, we challenge you to spend time on improving the sexual aspects of your relationship. If either of you is unfulfilled in your sexual relationship and you are not talking about it, then your marriage is currently in a state of crisis. This environment opens the door to resentment and anger, and even worse, the desire to look outside the marriage to meet those physical or emotional needs.

Based on patients that I see, women are seeking someone who will value them, protect them, and take care of them. There are deep-seated emotional needs. When those needs are met, it often leads to intimacy. For men, there is often a physical desire. If these needs are not met, temptation to meet these desires outside of the marriage often sets in.

There is never any excuse for going outside of your marriage to find sexual fulfillment. However, there are things that you can do for your husband or wife to make that sin less of a temptation; to remove its desirability. For men, start by listening to your wife; listen to her needs, hopes, and dreams. Be the caretaker of her emotions. Spend time communicating about intimacy. Find out what makes her feel sexually fulfilled. For women, make sure that you recognize your husband as the leader of your household. Be interested in the things that are important to him. Making a connection is important for true intimacy. Often times, though, making sure that you are actually having sex is enough to safeguard that part of your marriage.

As Paul says in his first letter to the Corinthians:

> The wife does not have authority over her own body but yields it to her husband. In the same way, the husband does not have authority over his own body but yields it to his wife. Do not deprive each other except perhaps by mutual consent and for a time, so that you may devote yourselves to prayer. Then come together again so that Satan will not tempt you because of your lack of self-control. I say this as a concession, not as a command. (1 Corinthians 7:4-6, NIV, 2011)

Questions:

1. Other than reading this book, are you spending enough time in communication specifically about your sex life?
2. What needs for sex and intimacy are being met in your relationship?
3. What specific needs can your spouse meet to help safeguard your marriage?

24.

This is too Hard/How Important is it to You?

Staying married in a world that treats marriage like a disposable commodity instead of a sacred union is a tough order. Many studies have evaluated common causes of divorce. If you do an internet search, you will see a wide variety of opinions and polls, but there are common themes. Money is frequently cited, which may speak more to a lack of communication or mismatched goals. Several of the polls or articles also list two separate things that are likely the same problem – infidelity and sexual incompatibility.

I have had many patients that were divorced and told me it was because they were "incompatible." What they have gone on to explain is that their spouse's sexual desires were completely out of sync with their own. Often, at the heart of this is a lack of communication or lack of a willingness of each to lay down their own desires for their spouse or vice versa. Sometimes the men are frustrated that their wives seem to have no sex drive or regard for their sexual desires. There are times that it is actually reversed, and she wants to have sex and he does not. You have already read separate chapters to address these subjects.

The question at hand is, "How important is it to you?" Is your marriage – the covenant you made with your spouse and God – more important than your own needs and desires? If your spouse desires more intimacy and you have been unwilling to participate, is it worth the health of your marriage to lay down your own agenda and seek to please your spouse? If your spouse is trying to meet you in the middle but you are pressuring him for more, are you willing to take a step back and recognize the effort he is putting forth?

One of my favorite sayings is, "I have not arrived, but I have left." If you are beginning the journey toward sexual healing with your spouse, take a moment to appreciate how far you have come. We are often overwhelmed by thoughts of where we should be, when often we should praise God that we have made significant progress. He does not expect us to arrive at a place of perfect holiness on this earth – salvation is a process filled with leaps forward and steps back. He loves us where we are and desires to carry us beyond where we think we can go. At every step of the journey, it is wise to count the cost and remind ourselves that our commitment to God and our spouses is worth the sacrifice and the work.

We have all seen that cute elderly couple that has been married for more than sixty years. I have the privilege of taking care of many women who have spent more years married in life than not, and still love the man to whom they are married. One woman recently told me that the secret was having at least one good fight a day. She went on to say that the problem lies not in the disagreements, but in the decision to remain silent when we are hurt or don't agree. In going through this book, I am sure you have found areas where you and your spouse disagree. Praise God for your differences and work toward compromises you can both live with and build your future upon.

Questions:

1. Have you had times that you thought your marriage was over? What made you stay together?

2. Have you seen progress in your intimacy since you started taking time together? How far have you come? Take a moment to reflect on the areas that have changed for the better.

3. Tell your spouse what he or she has done in the area of intimacy that you appreciate.

CPSIA information can be obtained at www.ICGtesting.com
Printed in the USA
LVOW08s0038091015

457533LV00001B/6/P